Breast Cancer:

Treatment Options for Metastatic or Stage IV Breast Cancer

Dr Matilda Benjamin

Acknowledgement

I would like to extend my most heartfelt thanks to each and every member of the medical community as well as each and every researcher who has contributed their valuable time and knowledge to the study and treatment of breast cancer. This book would not have been written if it weren't for their diligent efforts. In addition, I would like to express my gratitude to the patients and survivors who have generously shared their own narratives and experiences, which have provided both helpful insights and motivation. In closing, I would like to express my gratitude to my family and friends for their unflinching support during the whole process of writing this article.

Contents

3

ADVANCED BREAST CANCER

I will be discussing advanced breast cancer, also known as stage four or metastatic cancer, in this book. I will discuss what advanced breast cancer is, the many treatment choices, and then a few very particular things you need to know regarding tests that should be done on the tumor.

The phrase "advanced breast cancer" is sometimes used interchangeably with "metastatic cancer" and "stage four cancer," although it refers to all stages of the disease. I will refer to the disease as advanced breast cancer throughout this whole book since I feel that this word is clearer.

Having advanced breast cancer indicates that the disease has gone to other regions of the body from the breast as well as the nearby lymph nodes in the armpit or even in the region above the collarbone. This can occur before you are even diagnosed with breast cancer.

Where cancer cells leave the primary tumor and spread through the bloodstream or the lymphatic system and sort of nestle into other tissues like the liver, the lung, or the bone. To be honest, there are very few places where breast cancer cells won't find a home, but I've just mentioned the most common places now. There are two ways that advanced cancer can be diagnosed: through a biopsy or a blood test. Now two ways advanced cancer can be diagnosed: through a blood test or The first and most common scenario is that a person receives treatment for their primary breast cancer. They may undergo surgery, radiation therapy, chemotherapy, targeted therapy, or hormonal therapy. Years later, the cancer comes back in other parts of the body. Does this mean that your treatment didn't work? No, it means that it just didn't work well enough. Without that treatment, the cancer may have come back sooner, so the treatment was not in vain. However, what you're facing is a situation in which the cancer has People can also be diagnosed with advanced cancer if, at the time of their diagnosis, it is discovered that they have the disease in other parts of their body. About one in ten women in the United States and worldwide will have stage four disease at the time of diagnosis. Since this condition is also known as ADVANCED BREAST CANCER, the information that follows will refer to both types of advanced breast cancer.

We don't yet have treatments that can cure advanced cancer, but I'm going to tell you about a small proportion of people who live many, many years with no evidence of advanced cancer. This is up to five percent of people who've been told they have advanced cancer that we can't cure, but in those women, including a patient and several patient survivors, the goal of treatment is to help you live as long as possible with as good a quality of life as possible. At this point, we don't have treatments that can

This indicates that if you feel worse while receiving therapy than you do when you are not receiving treatment, we need to make adjustments to the treatment plan.
I can't cure this, so I need to make you feel as good as possible. That's what you want to hear from your doctor. This can be difficult for doctors to talk about, and even patients who are told this sometimes have a hard time hearing it. You must talk with your medical team, you must ask questions and clarify, and you must make sure you are on the same page.
Therefore, you would expect anything like

that in reaction to such grave information.

TREATMENT FOR ADVANCED BREAST CANCER

How should we approach the treatment of advanced breast cancer? You'll have a pet cat perhaps or a cat scan and a bone scan, and then if we're not certain this is what it is, we would do a biopsy of the safest area at a biopsy. Why do we do that? well, the first thing we need to know is, where is it in the body you will find that if you are diagnosed with something like cancer that has recurred in the bone your team will order scans of your entire body, not your brain Sometimes, we discover a whole new kind of cancer or perhaps something that isn't cancer at all.

So the standard of care is whenever possible if we think that your cancer has spread to other parts of the body that you should have a biopsy of the safest and most fruitful area to biopsy now the biopsy results can take a while so be patient this is something that you can ask for even if it hasn't been done the other parts of your workup will be blood tests including tumor markers which we don't do in people who've been treated with an intent to cure but about half of women with advanced cancer will have elevated tumor markers, if they're elevated we can use them later on to see how you're responding so we've covered what is advanced cancer and how you should be evaluated if we think you have advanced cancer in the treatment of advanced breast cancer, we have many different treatment modalities we can use in general we think about HORMONAL THERAPY, we think about CHEMOTHERAPY, TARGETED THERAPY RADIATION and even surgery in some patients the treatment decisions are based on the tumor biology specifically is the tumor hormone receptor positive that is does it have the estrogen and progesterone receptor Another important aspect that we take into consideration is whether or if the tumor has her two positive.

If the tumor is positive for hormone receptors, then we will most likely employ hormonal therapy. You may be thinking that this treatment is less aggressive than others, but keep in mind that the goal of treatment in advanced breast cancer is to help you survive for as long as possible while feeling as well as possible. Clinical tests have shown that patients who undergo hormone treatment have a life expectancy that is equivalent to that of patients who first undergo chemotherapy.

Remember that we're going to keep you on each treatment for as long as it's working what if you got five years on hormonal treatment before we even had to consider chemotherapy you feel much more normal and can perform your daily activities the decisions that we use to decide on hormonal therapy, in general, the factors that we use to decide on hormonal therapy, in general,

the decisions that we use to decide on
hormonal therapy, in general, the factors
that we use to decide on hormonal therapy,
in general, the decisions that we use to
decide on hormonal therapy in general
If that's the case, we have another hormonal
treatment in mind for you to try.
In all candor, we also consider whether or
not you have gone through menopause.
Ovarian suppression is something that
should be considered if you are approaching
menopause.
Why do we do that? Because when we
suppress your ovaries, we reduce the
amount of estrogen that is generated by the
ovaries, and this gives us access to a much
wider range of alternatives. using a
treatment based on hormones hormone
therapy as a treatment for advanced breast
cancer, which, once again, is more tolerable
and effective to the same degree. For how
long do you plan to undergo hormonal
therapy?

If you have a good response, a durable response, which means that you respond for a long period—months or even years—when that treatment stops working, we reach for another hormonal therapy. However, now that we have so many options in hormonal therapy, what we generally do is start with one and see how you respond. I'll explain how we follow you in just a moment. But what we generally do is start with one and see how you respond.

Therefore, in most cases, an advanced disease What we want to do is start with one treatment and then go on to the next drug in the same modality. For example, we may begin with hormone therapy a and then move on to hormonal therapy b. However, at some point, the majority of breast cancers develop resistance to hormonal therapy. At this point, we consider chemotherapy and targeted therapy.

When endocrine treatment or hormonal

therapy isn't producing the desired results, we will talk to you about the possibility of undergoing chemotherapy. We tend to use two or more drugs together because what we're trying to do is give you yes, a lot of side effects but the goal is cure remember that I said the goal in metastatic or advanced disease is to help you live as long as possible feeling as good as possible we know from clinical trials that in most women one chemotherapy at a time followed by when that stops working is the most effective treatment plan.

chemotherapy in the curative setting is something that we've covered in another book.

In such cases, we will utilize a variety of protocols in conjunction with targeted treatment that is aimed at the two proteins. Therefore, if you have chemotherapy that we are unable to use in conjunction with Herceptin and it is one that you have never got, we will not use it on you since you need the Herceptin plus targeted treatment.

Now that we've discussed hormone treatment and chemotherapy, you may hear the phrase "single agent sequential therapy" used in medical settings.

There are, however, a few notable exceptions to this rule. If you have an advanced form of cancer that has a large tumor load, which means you have a lot of cancer in your body, doctors may occasionally mix two treatments since doing so helps them function more quickly. But this isn't usually the case any more thanks to targeted therapy; I've already brought up Herceptin, and I've also mentioned that there are new targeted therapies; it's important to note that the majority of targeted therapies are administered in conjunction with chemotherapy; not all of them, but the majority of targeted therapies are administered with chemotherapy, and they help the chemotherapy work more effectively. There are even some drugs where the chemotherapy and the targeted therapy are combined into a single medication; as medical technology improves, we update our treatment options

OVARIAN SUPPRESSION OR ABLATION

How long it's been since your last treatment, whether or not that treatment will work again, and particular features of your tumor now I'm going to talk about one particular type of hormonal therapy which is ovarian suppression or ablation, in some women this alone can lead to regression of cancer the tumor can respond just to having your ovaries suppressed with shots or removed surgically, and although it's less common in this country, radiation therapy over just five days can kill cancer cells. ovarian suppression or ablation

TREATMENT
NOW I'M GOING TO TALK ABOUT SPECIFIC medication TO SPECIFIC SITES

IN THE BODY IF YOU HAVE ADVANCED CANCER. So far, we've been talking about systemic therapy, which is a medication that travels through your whole system. Keep in mind that these cells have already gone via your circulation and lymphatic system to your liver, bone, and other organs.

What about certain locations where we often contemplate surgery for breast cancer? Why am I not talking about surgery yet? There are a few situations in which we could take into consideration performing surgical procedures. One is that if your diagnosis is made and you still have cancer in the breast, we are going to treat the rest of the cancer throughout your body because that is the priority. After all, that is the life-limiting disease, but sometimes we also see such a response in the breast tumor itself that if everything is going well you're responding to treatment and you have what we call a durable response lasting months or years, many women will be offered the chance to remove the breast tumor itself. This is the case if you have what we call

It is psychologically beneficial, as it can help you feel like you are doing everything possible, and also why not treat it while it's responding, so first things first your whole system, and then we think about the breast the key things to know is that if treatment is working throughout your whole system, it is also working in the breast when wouldn't, we do surgery for somebody with a breast tumor still there who has advanced disease well, in some women the disease in the breast is advanced before the disease spreads to other parts of the

Do not feel as if we have given up on you if surgery is not indicated; rather, it is because you are doing so well without the need for surgery. a few more factors, including severe illness and the need for surgery These are particular circumstances that might or might not apply to you. For example, if you have cancer in the bone—for example, in the femur or the long bone of the leg—and there is an area that is painful or that is at risk for a fracture—we call this a pathologic fracture because it's due to the pathology of the tumor—you might have surgery to stabilize that bone, followed by radiation therapy. This is a very serious event.

However, the operation is connected with a short period needed for recuperation and the radiation treatment that comes after it is also completed in a relatively short period. The second situation in which we could recommend surgery is if you have cancer that is pushing on your spinal cord. While this kind of disease is often treated with radiation before surgery, there are certain patients for whom surgery is the most effective course of treatment. Other ideas may be anything like a region If the cancer is, for example, developing around the lung and you are experiencing fluid buildup around the lung, we will perform a procedure to help keep the lung open. This procedure is not technically considered surgery because it is performed by interventional radiology; however, it is still considered to be another procedure. Rarely, people will experience a recurrence of breast cancer in the brain; however, for many patients, surgery is necessary, and in general, radiation is used.

RADIATION

Next, I'm going to talk about radiation I've already mentioned that we might use that in treating the bone after surgery, but radiation is extremely effective in treating symptoms related to advanced cancer I'd say the

 The most common scenario in which I've recommended radiation therapy is in people who have painful bone lesions. Radiation therapy is nearly 100% effective with a very short course of radiation.

We're talking about 10 treatments. Some people can even be treated with one treatment. Can you imagine you have pain in a rib or your back or your shoulder? We can treat this with one treatment.

 So this is an option for you even if the cancer is responding to your systemic treatment sometimes we'll want to radiate that bone lesion because it's either severe or it's causing a lot of pain so radiation is good for treating symptoms it doesn't go through the whole body other situations would be if you had breast cancer on the chest and it was bleeding radiation therapy works incredibly well for that without surgery there's some other situations as well in which radiation therapy can be indicated and your yerba report will let you know if that's an option for you but don't think radiation therapy is ruled out because this is a systemic disease finally the last thing I'd like to cover is bone directed therapy for people who have bone metastases cancers in the bone the standard of care is to give what we call bone-directed therapy.

This is a medicine that you get to strengthen the bone interestingly enough we use these medications to treat osteoporosis you might know of Boniva which we see advertised for osteoporosis or Phoenix and you may even have been on one of these medications or maybe on it now the problem with these medicines given for osteoporosis is we don't absorb them enough once you have disease in the bone we'd like to give this through your system, not like chemotherapy or targeted therapy this is much more of a maintenance or preventative therapy but interestingly enough these drugs reduce pain to reduce the risk of fracture reduce the need for surgery and have very few side effects which I'll cover in just a moment.

TYPES OF BONE DIRECTED THERAPY
There are two major types of bone-directed therapy one are bisphosphonates and these are given now every three months it used to be monthly but we know every three months is just as good and you will stay on this medication for as long as you have bone involvement and there are no side effects.
 The other type of medication is called a rank ligand inhibitor which is spelled over

here these medications are primarily denosumab other ones are being developed of course the brand name is Exgiva and if you've been on prolia for the management of osteoporosis it's the same medication they just renamed it for different reasons for different uses this medication can be given under the skin, so if you don't have a port a semi-permanent IV and your IV is really difficult to get you can get these medications under the skin now these are difficult to get covered by insurance because they're very expensive so we restrict these for just a few people who can't tolerate the bisphosphonates or people who don't have an IV.

SIDE EFFECT
I said i'd talk about the side effects the bisphosphonates can cause aches and pains until we get the bone disease under control and for the first couple treatments you can actually get a flu-like syndrome this goes

away so don't give up you'll get it with possibly the first treatment we see this about one in five people, so four out of five people don't have this flu-like syndrome occasionally people can get it with the second treatment most people just get it with the first so try to stick that out because these medications are really a key part of managing bone involvement a very rare side effect of the bisphosphonates is something called OSTEONECROSIS of the jaw you don't even need to know what that is to find that quite alarming basically we see that areas in the bone won't heal so if you have a dental procedure it's possible like if you have a tooth removed that area may not heal people who are at risk for this complication are people who smoke who don't have great care of their teeth at the beginning or who actually it's actually kind of random but in general it's quite rare what we recommend is before we start bisphosphonates you see your dentist have any work done that needs

to be done invasive work like removal of
teeth etc and then you follow with the
dentist fairly oftenNwe don't have a lot of
preventative strategies right now for
osteonecrosis of the jaw but there are
several drugs and clinical trials we'll keep
you updated in theNfuture.

 If that happens we don't see the side effect
with the rank ligand inhibitors the biggest
side effect of the rank ligand inhibitors is
something called fragility fractures which is
not so much a concern in people with
advanced disease where we're treating
known disease in the bone it's more of a
concern in somebody who might be getting
preventive therapy for osteoporosis and the
other side effect, of course, is the cost and
that's a very real thing for most people.
 So I've covered what advanced cancer is.
I've covered treatment options.

GOAL OF TREATMENT

what the purpose of the therapy is intended
to be If you've been treated in the adjuvant
setting, you may not have been seen by your
oncology team for a while, and you may be
wondering what it will be like in general in
people with metastatic or advanced disease,
we see whenever you're on treatment the
frequency varies, but you're seeing either
every chemotherapy cycle or if you're on
hormonal therapy, we'll see you every three
months or so once we know the treatment
schedule. the last thing I'd like to cover
What about scans? Well, in the early stage of
breast cancer, when we treat it to cure it, we
don't conduct scans since they don't tell us
anything. However, if you have symptoms in
the advanced condition, we do scans.
However, we have measurable disease we've
seen it on a cat scan or a bone skin or a pet
scan or even on an x-ray so we'll follow

those exact same scans we try not to switch it up and do a different test we use the same test that identified the cancer and we do those scans in the beginning pretty much every three months after you're in a partial remission or maybe even a complete remission will follow you less often the key thing is to know that if you have symptoms that schedule falls apart and we will see you and evaluate you and see if you need to have a change in treatment just because the cancer may have started growing again doesn't mean there aren't any options at some point people with advanced cancer will have been a situation where further anti-cancer treatment causes more harm than good and it's important to know that you're part of that decision as well so in people where their cancer has not responded to three treatments we generally start talking about what's called maximal supportive care or aggressive symptom management.

If you are not qualified to participate in a clinical trial, our advice would be for you to educate yourself on the many alternatives available to you. Other options include the management of your symptoms, and in fact, you'll feel better off of chemotherapy. I've had patients who didn't want to stop chemotherapy, and when I suggested that we take a break, they called me a month later and said, "I haven't felt this good in years." This tells me that we haven't been achieving our goals, and the second thing is that they're going to get a better quality of life by being on palliative care or hospiceIt's incredibly essential that you maintain lines of communication open, questions like "why am I being treated" and "is the treatment working." We'll address this issue in another video because it's kind of a large topic to think about, but you must do it.

You can ask your doctor what will I do if

this doesn't work, and they'll say well it will work, and you can say I think so too If it doesn't how many other options do I have so be brave, you will find that you have more power the more knowledge you have, and make sure you get support from other people. What's next, in my notes, I always say if this doesn't work, this is my next plan. Make sure you have faith in your doctor to provide you with truthful information, but they also need to know that's what you want. By telling them that, you're essentially permitting them to be truthful with you. Boy, have we covered a lot of ground, and this is pretty heavy stuff. I wish you didn't have to go through this, but I do believe that knowing gives you power, so if this was helpful, please stay in touch with our medical books and share them with others so that they can benefit. This helps expand the reach of what we're doing for other people, and in the comments section, as I mentioned earlier, please let us know what else you'd like to learn about. I enjoy talking with you about what you're going through and how we can assist you.

Maintain your good health and safety.

www.ingramcontent.com/pod-product-compliance
Lightning Source LLC
Chambersburg PA
CBHW060019300526
45794CB00003B/1221